Nicky
Teaches her friends how to

Wash, Wash, Wash your hands

Written and illustrated by Evelyn Justiniano

Hi

My name is Nicky and I'd like to teach you and help you understand the importance of washing your hands.

When you properly wash your hands you can help prevent germs such as bacteria and viruses from spreading.

Bacteria and viruses can cause serious complications especially in children, the elderly and those with weak immune systems who are very vulnerable to illness.

By washing your hands properly with soap and water you remove germs and it helps prevent infection.

We tend to touch our eyes, nose and mouth with out even realizing we're doing so.

Germs can be transported threw the body by touching our eyes, nose and mouth and this can make us very sick.
This is why we must wash, wash, wash our hands.
Washing our hands is the first line of defense to stop many illnesses.

First you must wet your hands with water.

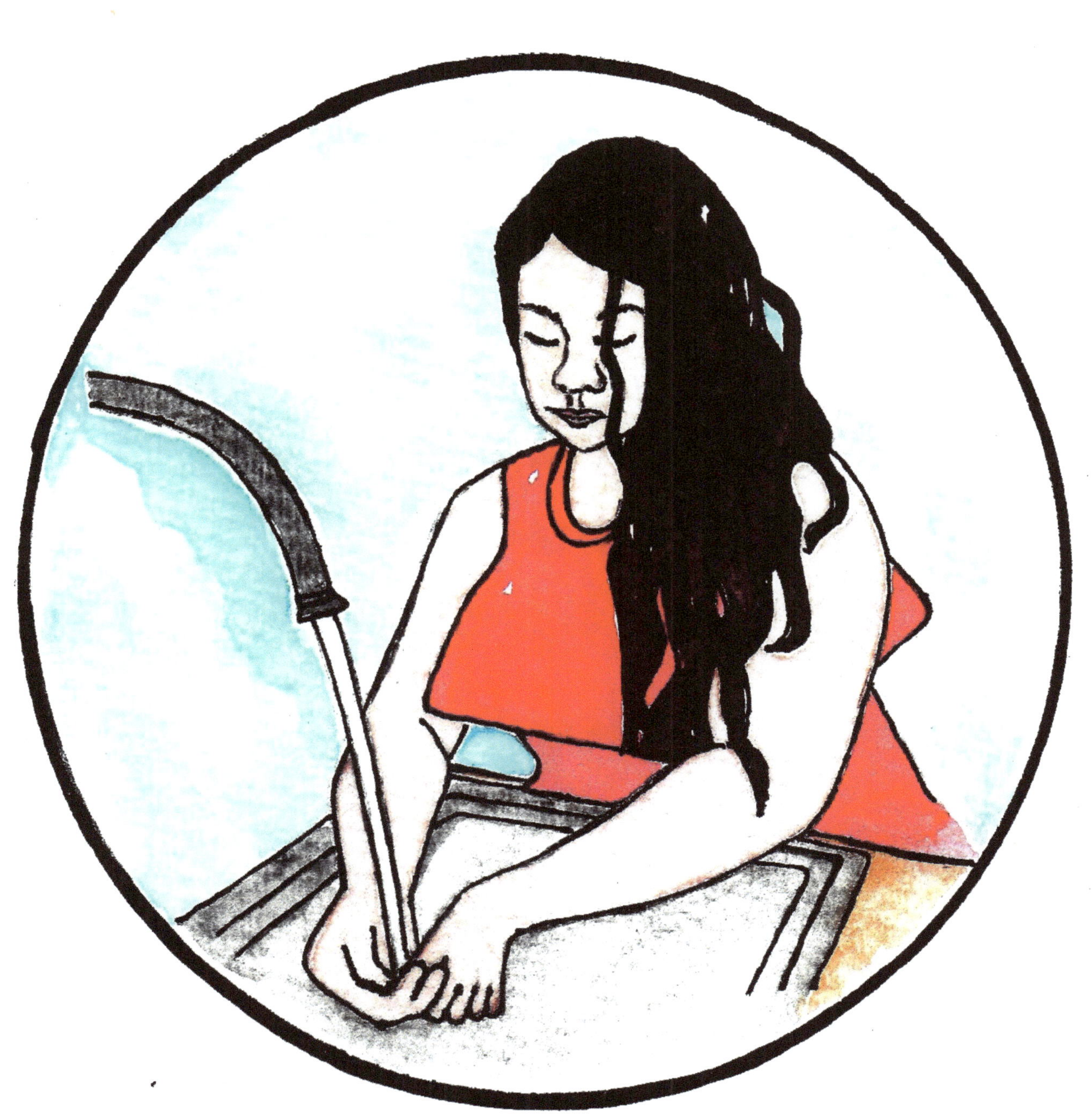

You must apply a generous amount of hand soap, about a dime or even quarter size.

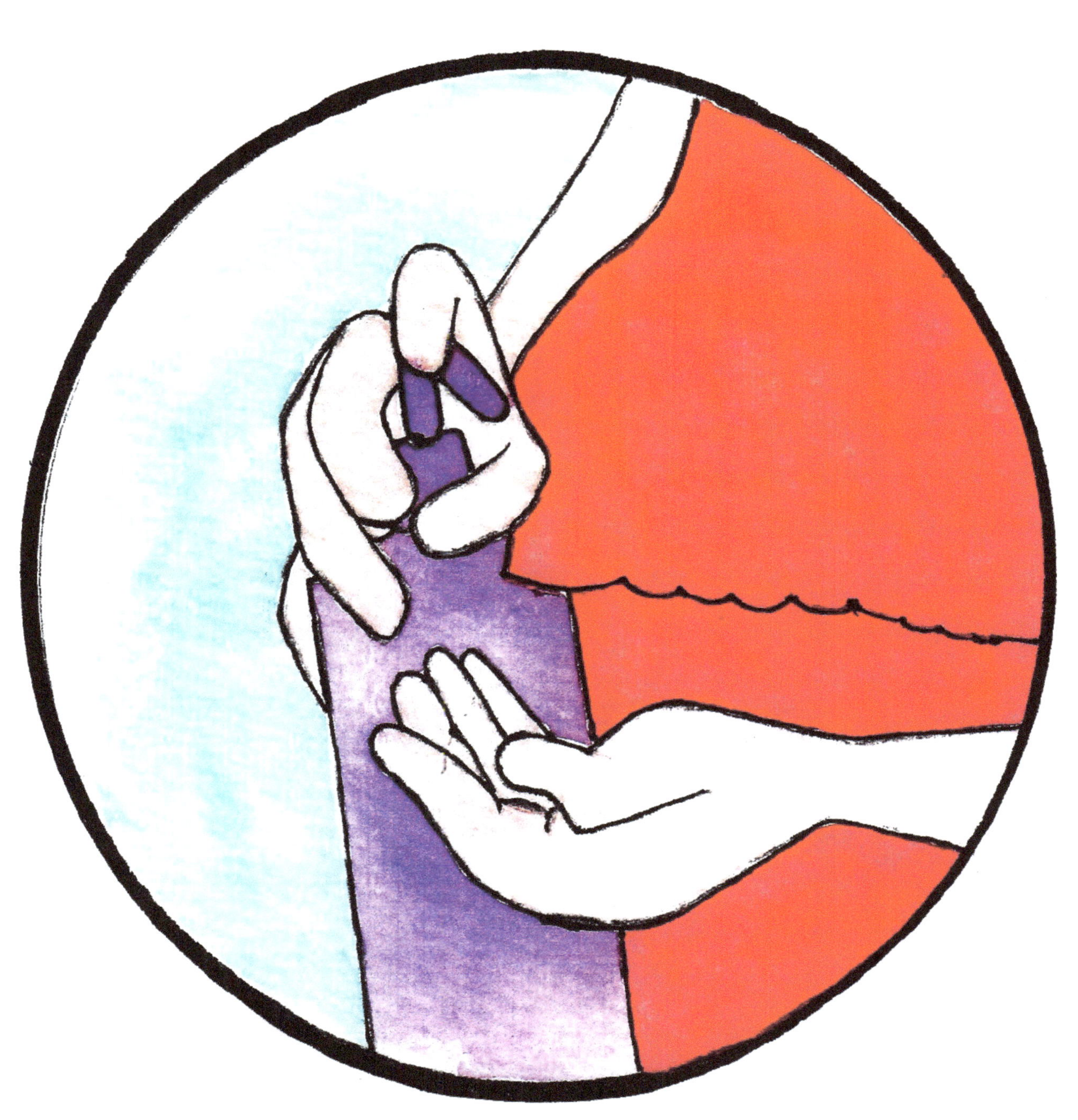

You must rub hands from palms to palms.

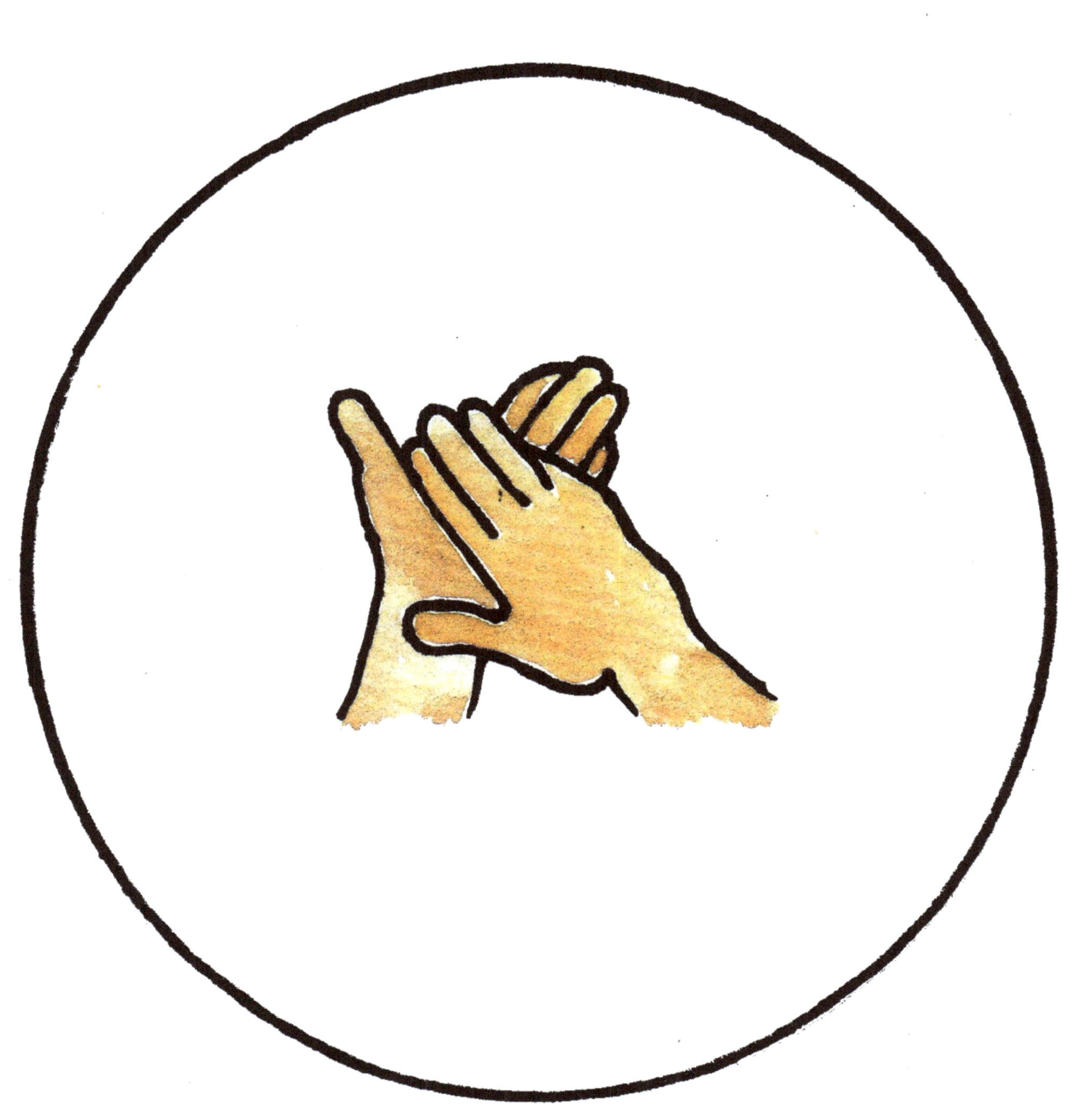

Use your right palm crossing over your
left palm.

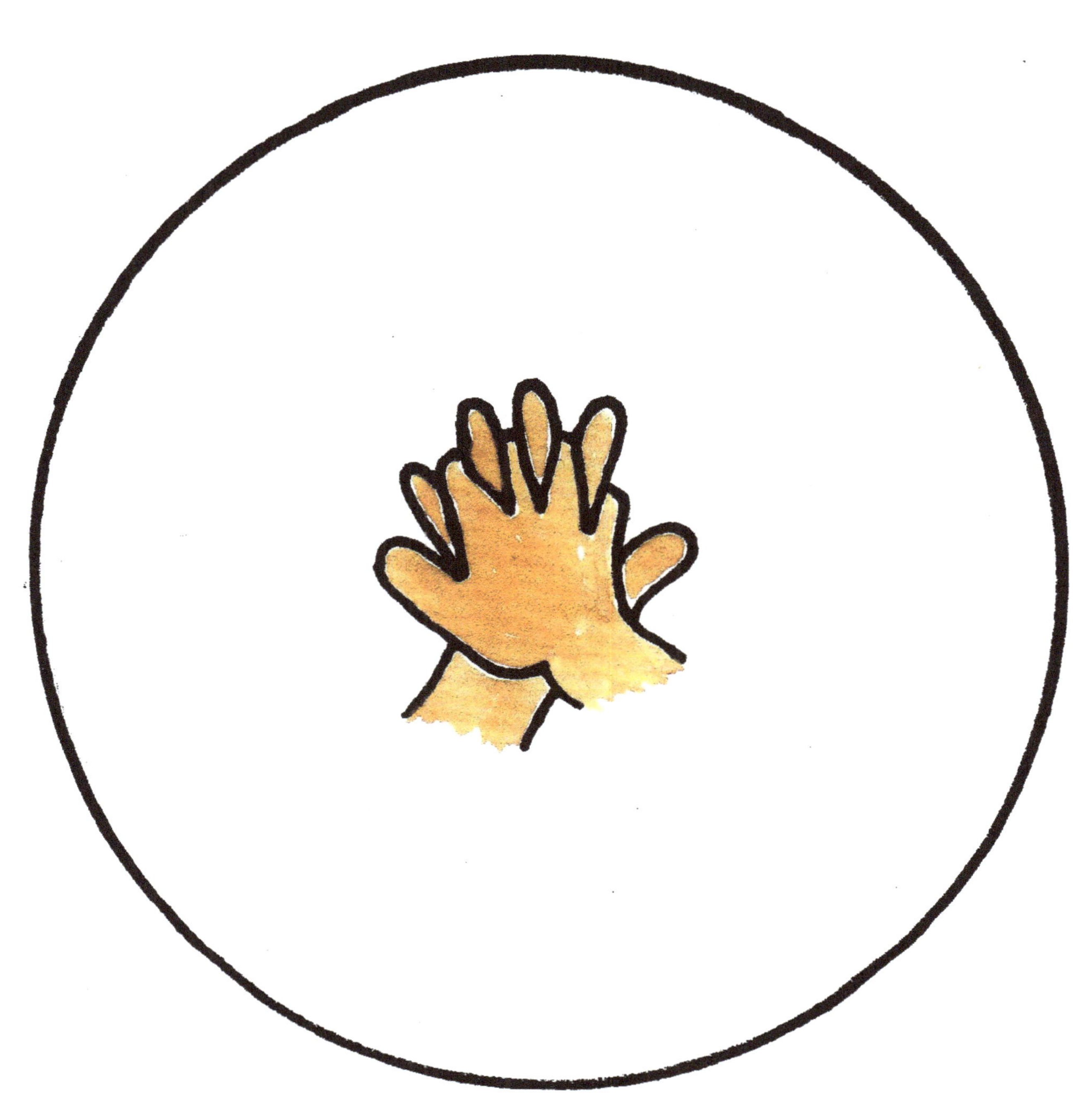

Then your left palm crossing over your
right palm.

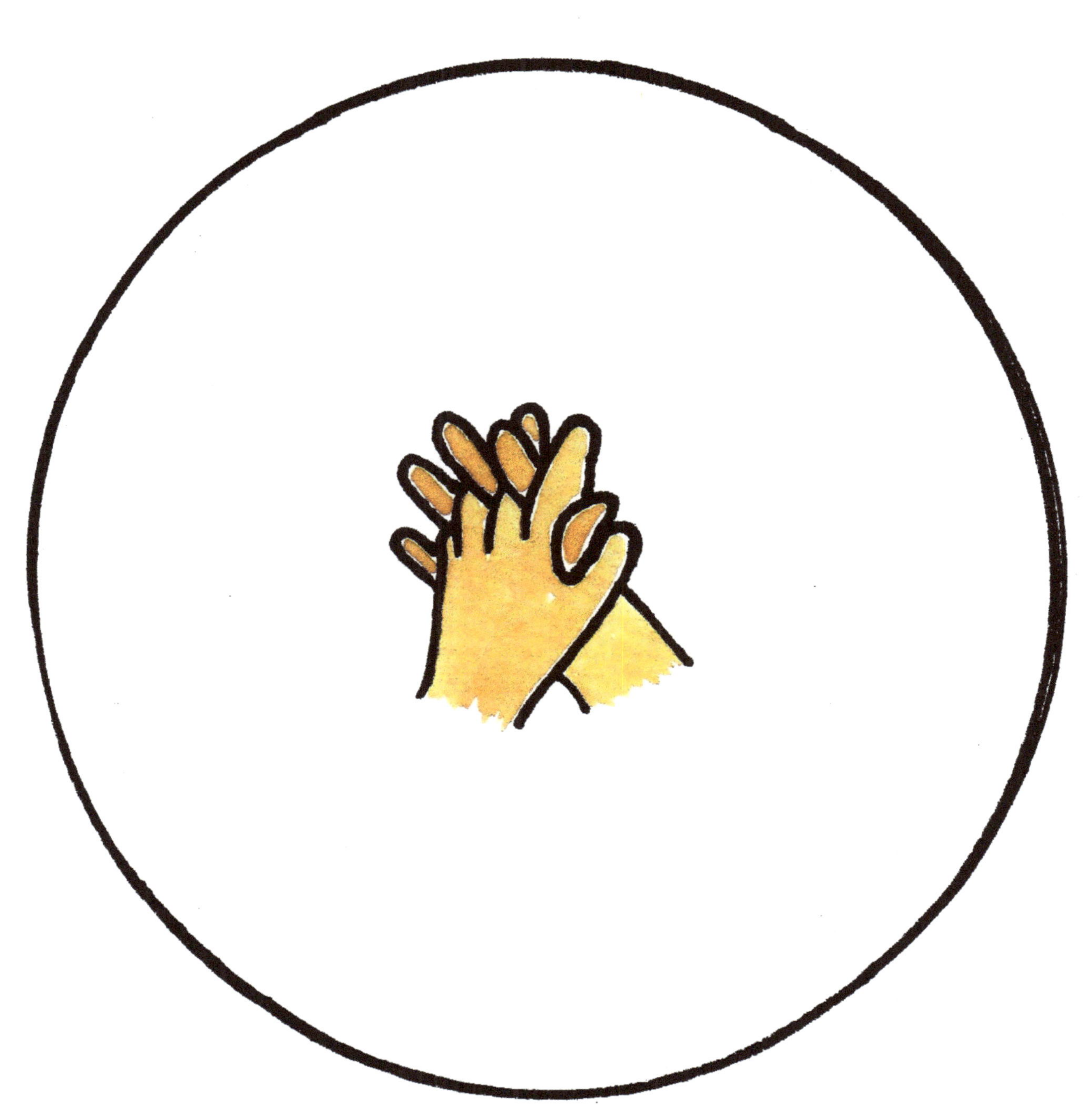

From palm to palm interlacing your fingers.

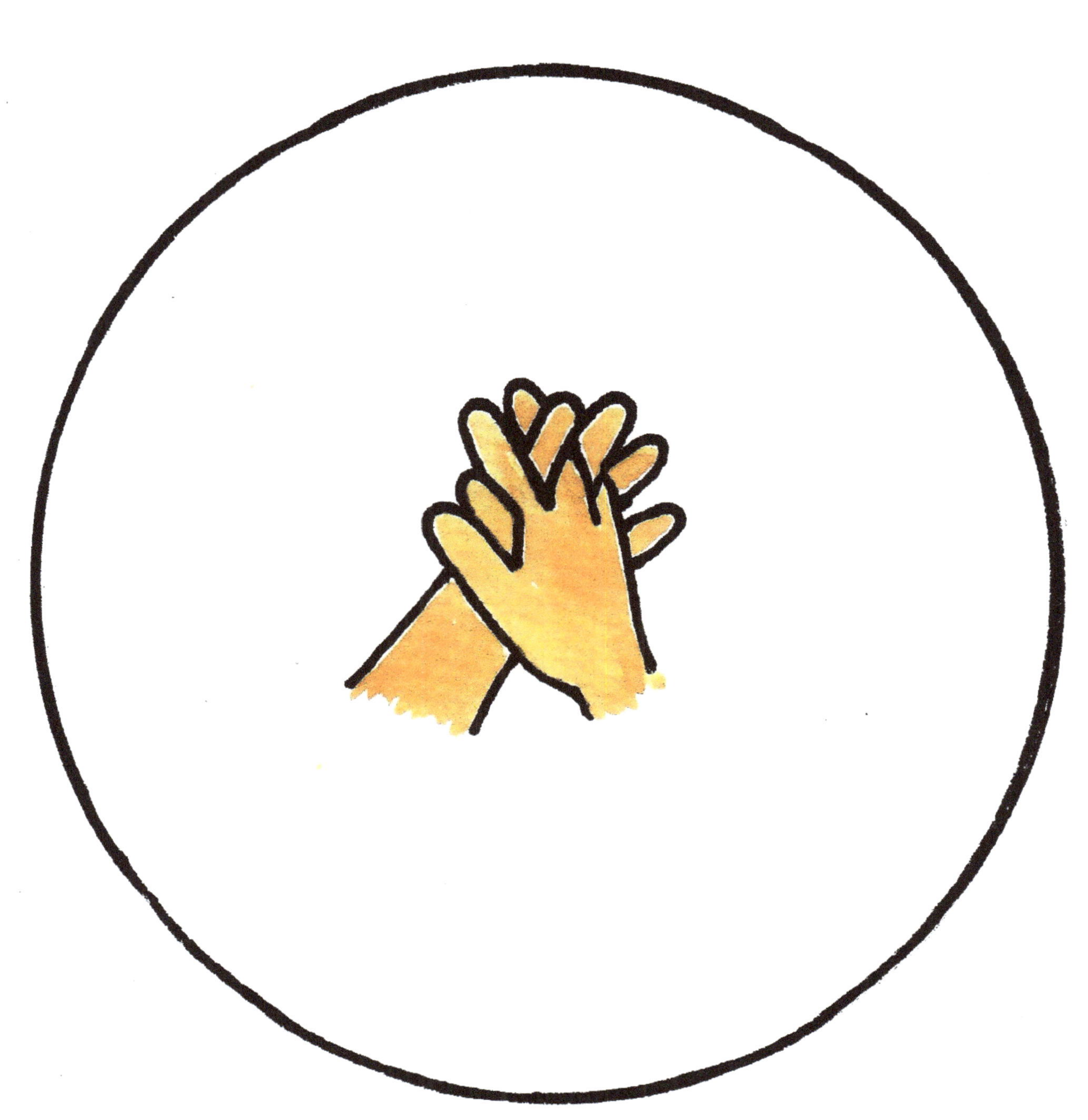

Then place the back of you fingers
opposite into your palms and interlock
while moving up and down.

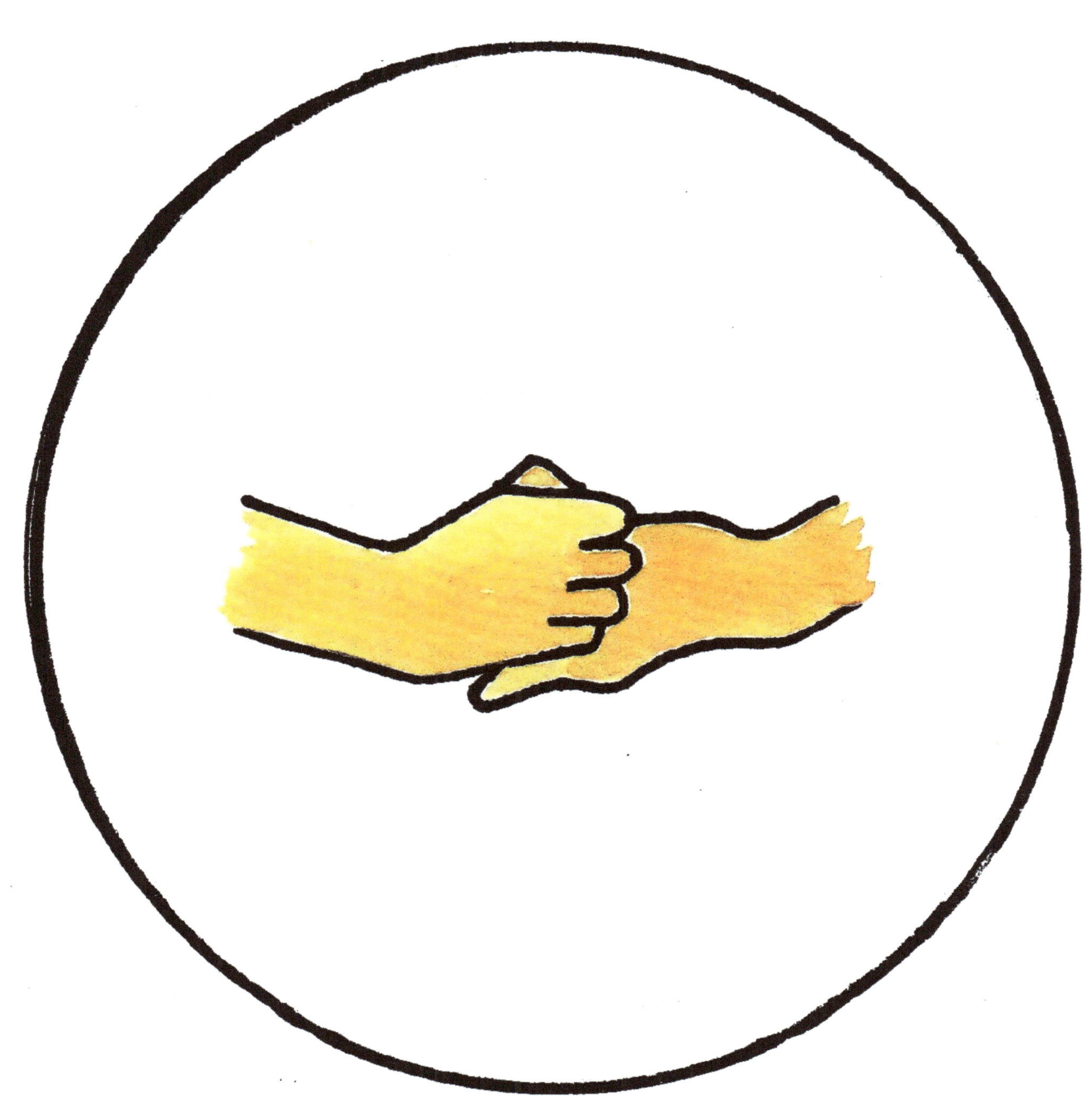

Then proceed to rub your left thumb within your right thumb.

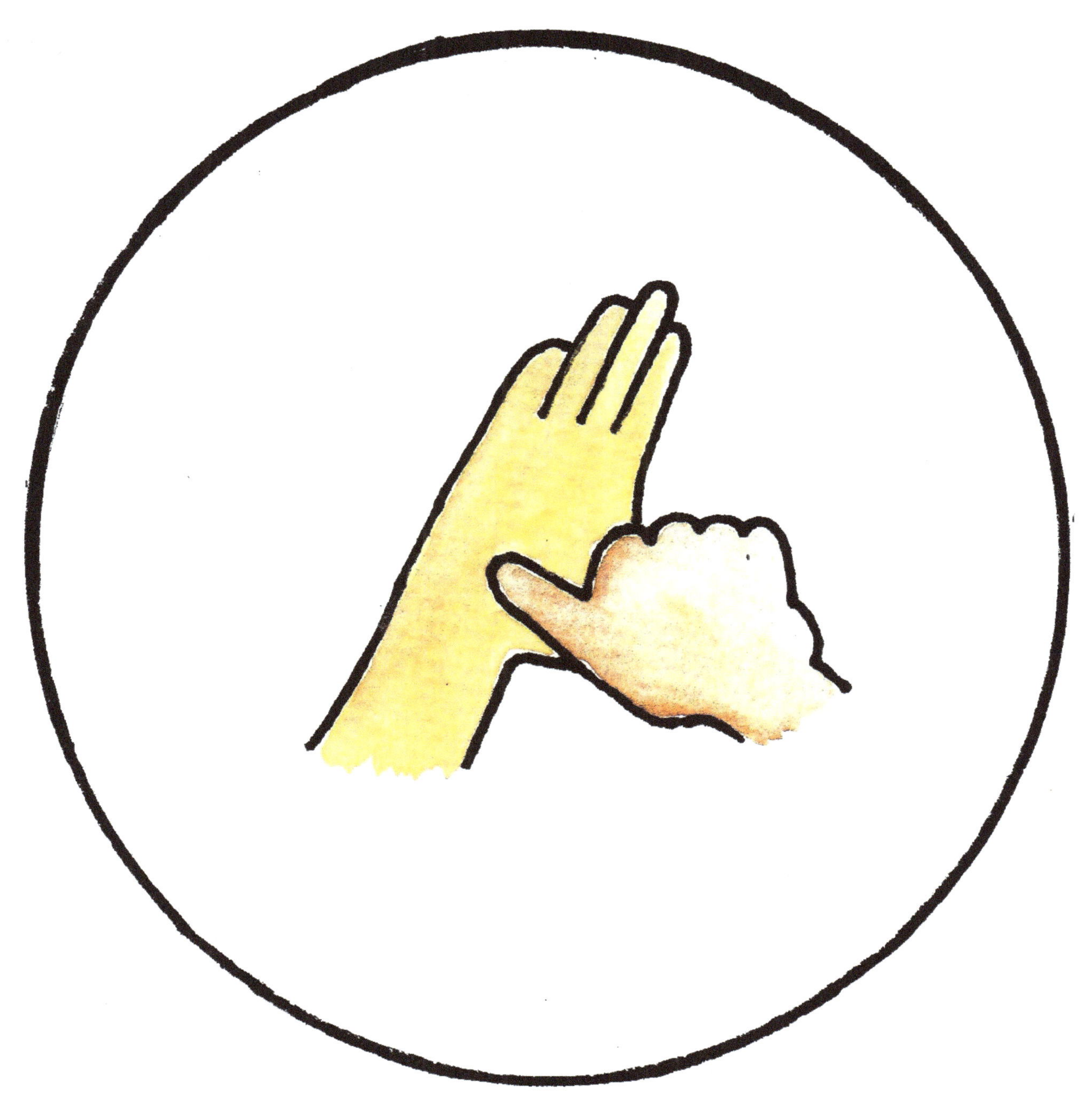

Next rub your right thumb within your
left thumb.

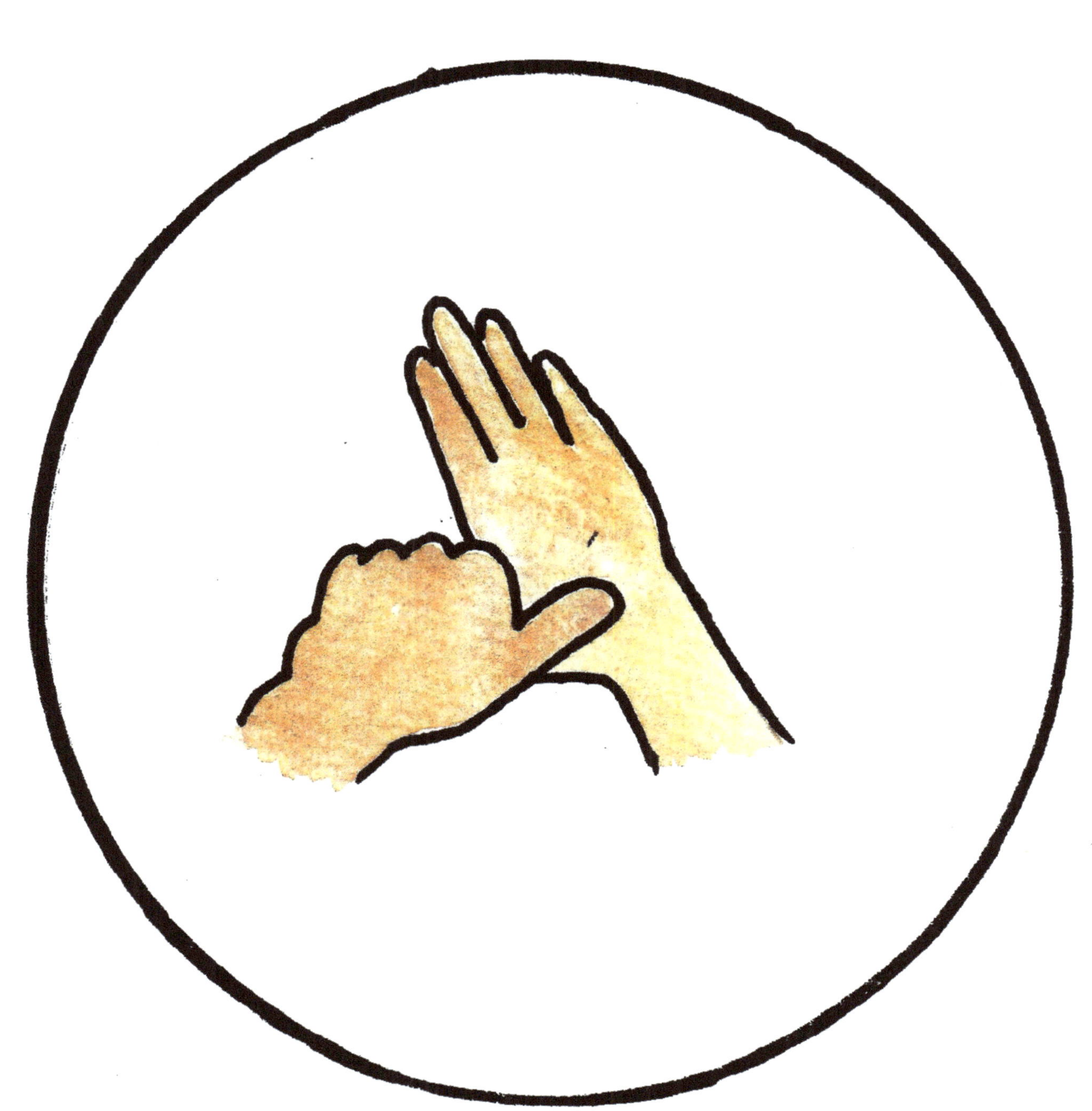

Then in circular motion with the tips of
your fingers scrub your right then your
left palms.

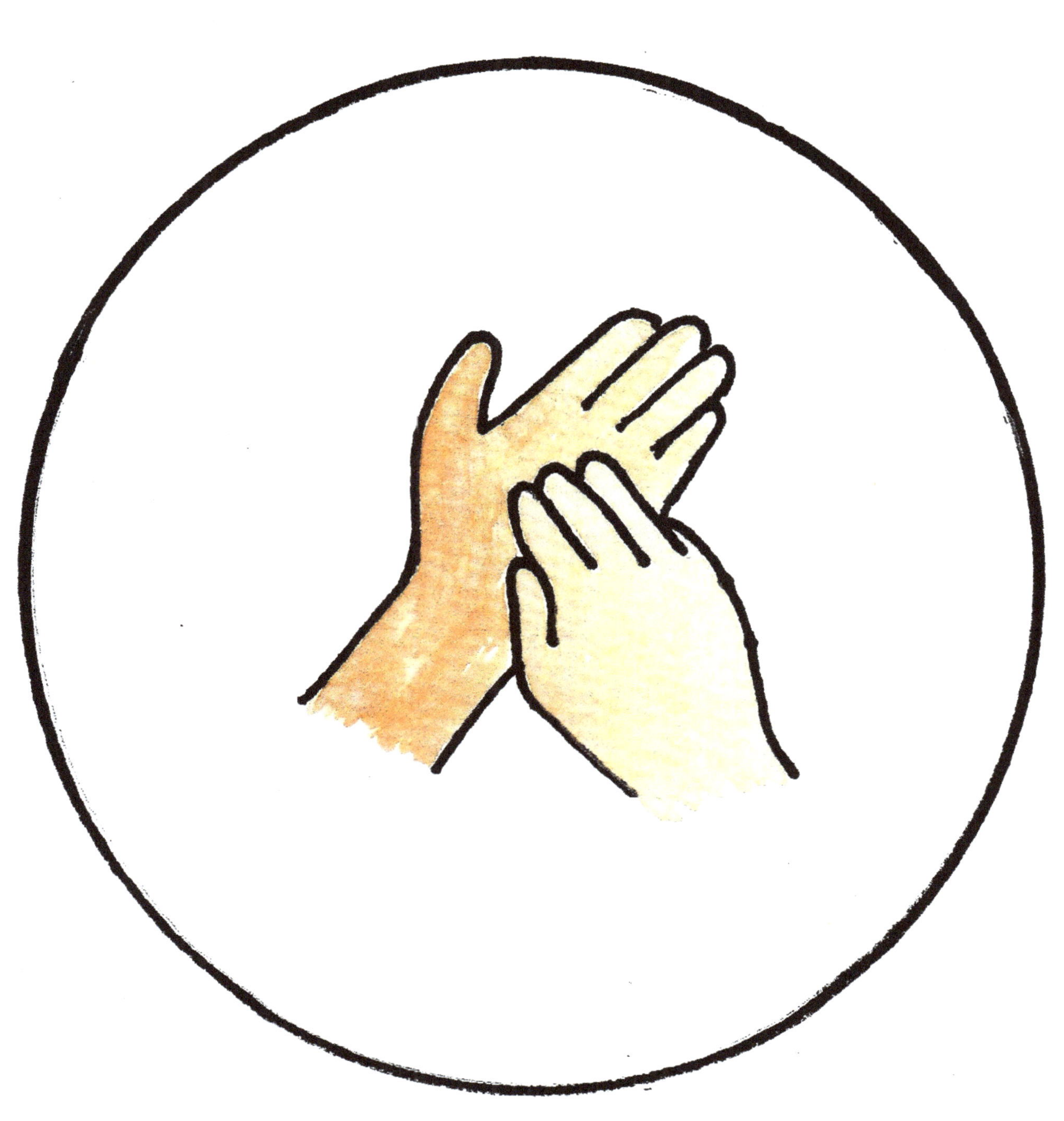

Next rinse your hands with warm water.

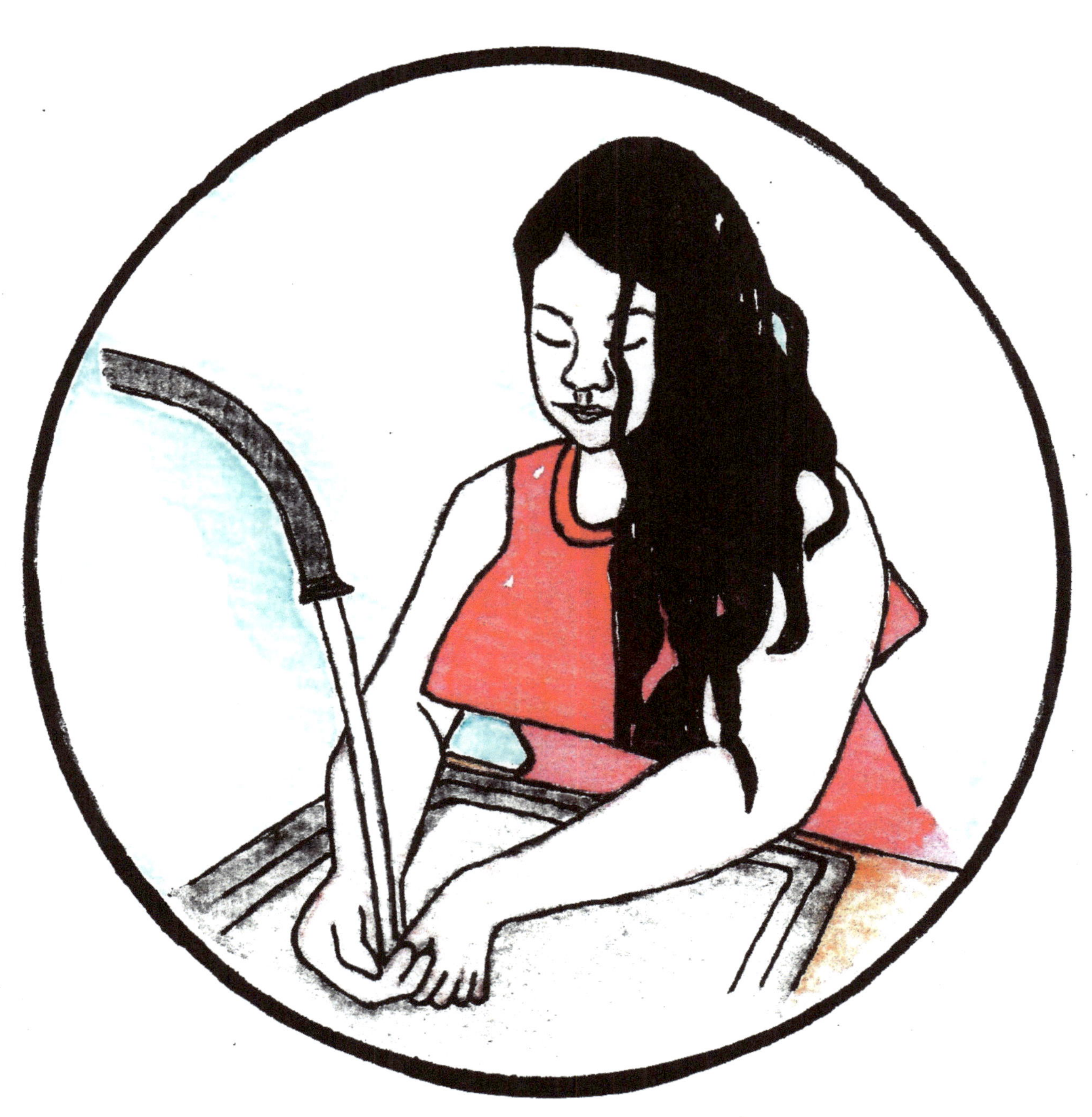

You are done.
Now you must dry your hands
thoroughly with an single use hand
towel.

Your hands now are clean.